I0464613

Hemodialysis From a patients view

By Robert Thomas

On Dec. 28th of 2011 I whined to Kaiser for a routing blood test a few days later I get this call on wed. From the doctor there were some problems with some blood work that they took I ended up at Kaiser Hospital for two days. I came home they didn't know why my kidneys were not doing their job. I went to see a specialist the flowing Thursday. It didn't look good; the Doctor put me on a vegetarian diet for all most a year. On Feb 22, 2012

I when'd and seen UCF Medical Center for Transplantation Evaluation see my Link page to see what they do. On March 1, 2012 I saw the Doctor for pre-surgery on March 5th I had my surgery for my fistula to be put in for Dialysis.

This is form a life story taken out of the Awake1/8/1985 * ("I eventually I would have to be connected with a kidney machine. This meant having two minor operations called fistula shunts—a process in which a vein is enlarged. This makes it easier to insert the needles used in kidney-machine treatment (haemodialysis). The first fistula shunt was not successful"

Haemodialysis is a fascinating process. First two needles are inserted into the veins. A peristaltic pump draws blood through one needle and several feet of connecting tube into an artificial kidney. This kidney does the actual cleansing of the blood. From there the blood passes through yet more plastic tubing to the second needle and thence back into the body. The kidney machine itself simply monitors the job.

The use of needles was, and still is, something quite difficult to endure. It is painful and sometimes takes several attempts. This is because the needle must go *along* a vein, threading it, as it were, and not *through* it. When this does happen, blood escapes, filling the surrounding tissue and causing a painful swelling, or bump. Then there were the problems of adjusting mentally and physically to the routine.")

For next ten days I was off work and sitting at home. The vegetarian diet was working for about a year. And then do to changes on the job on September 18th 2012 I was put on Hemodialysis. There are 2 types of Dialysis, Hemodialysis and (PDA) Peritoneal dialysis. So now I had chronic kidney disease (CKD), or kidney disease for short. Why did I choses Hemodialysis.

My circumstances did not allow for me to do (PDA) Peritoneal dialysis at home. And I was more comfortable with having someone hook me up to a dialysis machine. This is funny because I don't like needles. You can have a stent or a fistula. I was more comfortable with a fistula then a stent. Some treatment facility you can stay overnight and they do offer (PDA) Peritoneal dialysis at the treatment facility

Note * the information came from the watchtower bible and track society of Pennsylvania

This Awake 1/8/1985 **Alive! With the Help of a Kidney Machine**

My First Day and Week

I came to Satellite Dialysis the first thing I did was meet with the staff, I First meet with the a social worker she when'd over my Patient's Right's and ask me what my favorite activates were, and if I was working or not. how important it was to keep busy.

She helped me with my transportation needs, we when'd over how dialysis machine worked. I told her I didn't drive or have a car so my social worker gave me The Phone Number of paratransit. What is paratransit is a bus that helps disabled people get to Their appointments. And you may get the City Bus for free check your local city to find this out .Your social worker will help you with all and any need you may have**.**

Dietitian worker

She when'd over my new Diet and some Change's I would have to make She asked if I was on any medication, vitamins I was taking, and what my past Diet was like If I had a do over I would have made a list

1: all medication.

2: all vitamins or supplements

3: a list of food that I had been eating for the last 3 months

She told me how imported it is to stay away from high Potassium, Phosphorus foods.

She gave me a list of food to stay away form, also gave me a list of low Potassium, Phosphorus foods And a cook book to. Both your dietitian and Social worker will help you and answer all and any question you may have .They are there to help you and there are no stupid questions. **You must be you own advocate** and have someone come with you; they may come up with questions that you didn't think of or consider. Both your dietitian and Social worker will evaluate you every year on the date you first came in Ask your dietitian about Renal Meals form Council on Aging

Going into my first week

The Nurse will ask you about all and any surgery you may have had. The Hemodialysis technician Will try to determent what you dry weight is. And later will try to challenge your dry weight. Some Can take there dry weight being challenge. Others like me cant. You may get a different Hemodialysis technician every time you come in for treatment. **You must be you own advocate** remember the Nurse. And Hemodialysis technician are very busy and are working on other patients. If they have an Emergency or some patient may need a little more care. **You must be you own advocate**

Tell the Nurse and Hemodialysis technician of any problems you may have had with your Treatment or non-treatment Days. If you have any pane in the chest call 911 and on your Next Treatment let the nurse and Hemodialysis technician know. Later that week I learned that if you don't like needles have a good breathing technique is a good Idea why you may ask I pass out the second day I was there.

So when the needles are going in, breathe in Very deeply and let it all out keep doing this in tell Hemodialysis technician is done. All so you may bring worm closes after all you are sitting there for a long time you may get Cold, for the first year I wore thermals, all so you may bring a blanket and a pillow. Some patients sleep, watch T.V, read, or play game on their lap tops or tablets.

A treatment Day

The first thing you do is wash your fistula and weight yourself then go to your chair you Will to see if you name is on the dialyzer this is where you will sit Give you weight to the Hemodialysis technician, the Tech will take a standing blood presser Then a siting blood presser. The Tech then will hook you up to the dialysis machine. The needles will sting a little and tell your fistula gets use to it, it's very important to Exercise your fistula to keep it healthy, after you get hook up by Hemodialysis technician. The Tech will monitor you. And you will form time to time need to check your access to see if it's leaking or not if so let the Hemodialysis technician Or Nurse know right away.

Your blood presser will be monitored as well. The Hemodialysis technician Or Nurse will take your temperature. Once a month they will test your fistula to see how well it's working. Let the Hemodialysis technician Or Nurse know if you have any problems during the treatment, at the end of your treatment. You will take a siting blood presser and a standing blood presser. The Nurse will come up to you and check your Heart and lungs, all so she will inform you of all medication that she will be giving you during your treatment.

The Hemodialysis technician will disconnect you form the dialysis machine and pull your needles out and bandages up your access. Then you can hold the bandages or they can clamp them In tell your blood clots then you go and weight yourself and let the Hemodialysis technician know what your weight is then you're done!

Remember it's your health **You must be you own advocate** once a month you will have lab work done Every 3 month you will take a urine test. That is if you can urinate. This is all so how they determine how much liquids you can have. The less you can urinate the more restricted the fluids are. And your dietitian worker will go over all your lab work with you. Remember there is No stupid questions this is your Health **You must be you own advocate**

It will be a new lifestyle and maybe a hard journey

Even though you may be exhausted, fatigued, tired this will affect everyone differently remember to be kind to yourself while you process this. Learn all you can and take control, be your own advocate and don't let the disease manage you, YOU! Manage the disease

How to handle friend and family,

We all have friends and Family; unfortunately having a chronic health issue for some people who don't have a chronic health issue, have a hard time really understand what you're Dealing with so they may stop talking to you or coming around, they may not Want to see you go thru your chronic health issue or see you die this can be hard On some people

They may pretending there is no health issue or just avoid you. Every one reacts differently. Losing your friends and support is hard enough and being ill at the same time. This can be devastating. This is why it very imported to have a support system! I found my support system online.

To help are family and Friends to understand hear an illustration Ask your family & friends if they ever had the flu, when they say yes Ask them if they felt like doing their favorite activity, going to work having Friends and family over for dinner and a movie, they will most likely say no Ask them why don't you? They will say I would not be filling well, and then you can Say ok try filing like That 365 day of the year. They will get it.

You may be asking will I be able to maintain the same lifestyle that IM use to. Continue, try to keep active Live as normal as your body will allow you don't let dialysis define you. Go out enjoy being with your friends and family or doing what you like to do.

Hobbies

Keeping busy with everything not related to CKD or dialysis, having a hobby is a good idea. Things to do, Sewing, Cooking, shooting at a rang, video Games, taking up a craft and there many Types of Crafts, reading, creative writing, puzzles, Paint, restore furniture, photography, My Favorite things are video Games, reading, creative writing, photography.

Can I work?

Yes you can and many do. I worked for the first 4 months on Dialysis I was a janitor at a local Mall, I had worked there for 14 years and liked it a lot, and after I started Dialysis I was just too exhausted to finish my shift. So on Dec 31, 2012. I left and Whined on disability,

I started the paper work a few months or so before leaving my job. So now you're on disability you would like to work some, you can make up to a certain dollar amount before they touch your disability. This is what you need to do. Call or go the offices of SSA, SSI, Medicare /medical and talk to them about working they will have more information on working while on Disability

Know Your Rights as a Worker

People on dialysis have rights under the Americans with Disabilities Act. Your employer may be able to make accommodations that help you stay employed.

http://www.dol.gov/whd/fmla/#.UME-i6w0V8E

http://www.ada.gov/cguide.pdf

http://askjan.org/

http://www.eeoc.gov/

Remember empower yourself by understanding your rights as an employee with kidney disease. Whether you need to take a leave of absence or to adjust your workspace, take steps to learn about your rights and how to exercise them.

Will my Diet change?

Yes, will need to watch foods that are high in Potassium, Phosphorus. I have made a food log so you have an idea of what to eat. All so the treatment facility will give you a cook book. You also can google it; I have a link on the link page Try to be balance in what you're eating it will show up in you lab work. Your dietitian will give you a list of High and low Potassium, Phosphorus foods. Over time you will eventually learn what and what not to eat with what ingredients, your dietician can help you with a Dialysis friendly diet.

Things to know

What is Dry Weight?

Answer: the term "dry weight" means the amount of body mass (weight) without extra fluid (water). This is why the Nurse will check you for edema or shortness of breath in which you may have water in your lungs, if you get a headache or cramps this could indicate that they have taken you blow your dry Weight.

What is Rinse back?

Answer: you will see a saline bag that is connected to the dialysis machine This is used to clear the lines of air be for your treatment, during your treatment you will get some to help elevate any cramping you may have after your treatment You will get some to return your blood.

That doses the Kidney do?

Answer: your kidneys are your body's filter; they all so regulate your body temperature. It's not unheard of to be cold when others are not.

Can you eat or drink when you're on dialysis?

Answer: Yes some do, but this may affect your Blood presser, or affect how much Liquids is being taken off you, so you're not getting to your true dry weight.

Will your food may taste different

Answer: yes you may get a metallic taste your taste buds will change, try foods with strong Flavors like chills, herbs, spices

Insomnia

Answer: Yes form time to time you may get Insomnia, what so do when this

Happens go for a long walk just be for going to bed, if this does not work

Try lying down and resting if this does not work, talk to you Doctor about

Sleep ads.

Your fistula

Answer: You will get bulges or bumps don't hide them use them to educate people about Kidney disease, once it stops working it will go down

Everyone has a unique fluid restriction all way's check with your dietitian or nurse to find out yours

Tips for limiting fluid intake

1 if you have is diabetes keep good control of your blood sugar

2 stay cool

3 drink clod liquids in place of hot liquids
4 avoid salt

5 use small cups and glasses to feel like your drinking more

6 sip, don't gulp

7 add bit of lemon juice to water and ice

8 limit coffee

9 use your beverage at mealtimes to take phosphate binder and any other medications that may be taken with food

10 take your medications with applesauce

11 limit soups

Tips for relieving mouth dryness

1 brush your teeth

2 rinse your mouth with cold mouthwash (don't swallow!)

3 suck on sugar free hard candy, especially sour candy

4 snack on cold fruits and vegetables

5 eat small amounts of frozen grapes, one at a time

6 suck on a lime or lemon

7 eat bread spread with margarine and sugar free jelly

8 suck on some ice

Why limit your fluids

1 Your heart may not have to work so hard

2 it may be easier to breathe

3 your blood pressure may be easier to control

4 dialysis treatments may be more comfortable for you

5 drink liquids that have no sugar

6 watch your salt intake

Exercise

It's very important, go to a GYM, if you can't, use you home as the GYM this is what I do. Do you have an upstairs and downstairs there is your Stairmaster, walk or run around the block, go to google and do a search on Home Exercise for more ideas. All so KQED Public TV has a home exercise show

Depression

Like all chronic Disease that can profoundly affect are life's Depression can

Come up and we may not want to go on

I found this great article in the Awake 4/2014 Why Go On—Three Reasons to Keep Living

1 "things change Consider four faithful people mentioned in the Bible who suffered

despair to the point of not wanting to go on." Rebekah, Mossed, Elijah, Job

Their Circumstances Changed"

2 There is Help

Prayer, People Who Car, and Professional Assistance

3 there is Hope

The Bible Teaches of Jehovah's Promise

For the complete article go to JW.org

We can be Happy How

I found this great article in the Awake 11/2014 Keys to Happy life

1 "Find Contentment

2 Be Resilience

3 Be Positive

For the complete article go to JW.org

Note * the information came from the watchtower bible and track society of Pennsylvania

For more information on this subject and any other subject of interest please go to JW.org

Looking at Food Labels, Serving Size

Always look at the Nutrition Facts

1 **Sodium**

Look at the "MG" not the %

Less than 2000 MG/day, and 600 for a meal, 200 for a snack

2 **Potassium**

May not be listed, if it's not it does not mean there is no potassium

Low 100mg or 3%

Medium 101-200mg or 3-6%

High 201-300mg or 6-9%

Very high 300mg or 15%

3 **phosphorus**

Low 50mg or 5%

Medium 51-150mg or 5-15%

High 150mg or 15%

Remember it not all listed so look at the ingredient list for the words with

"Phos" in them, and add phosphorus very easily add up to 1000mg a day

This is my Food log just for 1 month

I all so put how I was filling be for and after Treatment

And my weight, this just to give you an idea of what you can eat

March

1st

Breakfast: 3 eggs, 1 cup of oak brand hot cereal, 3 sausage, coffee 16 ounces

Lunch: skipped

Dinner: beans, rice, turkey, chicken, 21 ounces water

No Treatment felt good all day some energy

2nd

Breakfast: 3 eggs, 1 cup of oak brand hot cereal, 3 sausage, coffee 16 ounces

Lunch: Renal Meal: shepherd pie/ rice pudding, corn nibbles/seasoned butter green beans no drink

Dinner: turkey, potatoes, cauliflower, broccoli   21 ounces water

Treatment Day filling good have some energy be for I go in came home with some energy

79.1 KG home 76.6

3rd

Breakfast: waffle slam at Denny's 3 cups of coffee ate out

Lunch: pork & beans 21 ounces soda

Dinner: hamburger lettuce tomato cheese avocado, salad 21 ounces soda, ate out

No Treatment a little tired

4th

Breakfast: 3 eggs 1 cup of oak brand hot cereal, 3 sausage, coffee 21 ounces

Lunch: Renal Meal: south west pork, white rice, green peas no drink

Dinner: Renal Meal: Turkey/cranberry sauce, bread stuffing, cranberry cabbage 21 ounces water

Treatment day a little tired going in coming home very tired

79.0 KG after 76.4 KG

5th

Breakfast: 3 eggs, 1 cup of oak brand hot cereal, 3 sausage, coffee 21 ounces

Lunch: chicken, cauliflower, broccoli   21 ounces water

Dinner: chicken, cauliflower, broccoli   21 ounces water

No Treatment felt good some energy

6th

Breakfast: breakfast burrito, 2, 21 ounces coffees

Lunch Skipped

Dinner beef/barley stew, white rice, corn cob, 21 ounces water

Treatment day going in was a little tired coming home had lots of energy

Going in 77.2 KG coming home 76.4 KG

7th

Breakfast: 3 eggs 1 cup of oak brand hot cereal, 3 sausage, coffee 21 ounces

Lunch: skipped

Dinner: out to eat Chevy's Super Cinco,   Two enchiladas: 1 soft beef taco, 1 tamale, 2 margaritas

No Treatment today filling a little tired

8th

Breakfast: skipped

Lunch: hotdog, soda 21 ounces, Ate out

Dinner: hot/ spicy chicken, teriyaki chicken, rice, soda 21 ounces, ate out

No Treatment today filling very tired

9th

Breakfast: 3 eggs 1 cup of oak brand hot cereal, 3 sausage, 3 coffee 21 ounces

Lunch: renal Meal: asparagus risotto, green beans, blueberry peach cries, And 21 ounces soda

Dinner: renal Meal: Chinese 5 spice chicken fried rice squash medley

Treatment day a lot tired be for going in come home still very tired

79.5 KG going in/ going home 76.4 KG

10th

Breakfast: 3 Donets, coffee 21 ounces

Lunch: Chinese spice chicken, fried rice, chow main, beef 21 ounces soda, ate out

Dinner: Chinese sweet sower pork, fried rice, chow main, 21 ounces soda, ate out

Ate out

No Treatment today filling a little better still tired

11th

Breakfast: cold cereal, coffee 21 ounces

Lunch: renal Meal: oven fried chicken, coleslaw, noodle/lemon, No drink

Dinner: chili hotdog, 21 ounces, ate out

Treatment Day be for going and after I had some energy

Be for going in 78.7 KG going home 76.5

12th

Breakfast: skipped

Lunch: salad, 21 ounces soda

Dinner: 2 pizzas, 21 ounces soda, ate out

No Treatment felt great has lots of energy

13th

Breakfast: skipped, coffee 21 ounces

Lunch: renal Meal: chicken fettuccine, summer squash medley, green peas, water 21 ounces

Dinner: renal Meal: oven BBQ chicken thigh, corn niblets/seasoned butter, green beans

Treatment Day filling ok be for going in after coming home very tired and had headache

14th

Breakfast: skipped

Lunch: hamburger plan, 21 ounces soda

Dinner: mac and chess, beef

No Treatment today little tired

15th

Breakfast: 3 eggs 1 cup of oak brand hot cereal, 21 ounces coffee

Lunch: skipped

Dinner: hotdog, tacos, 21 ounces water, ate out

No Treatment today some energy

16th

Breakfast: 3 eggs 1 cup of oak brand hot cereal, 21 ounces coffee

Lunch: Renal Meal: Cajun oven fried chicken, Cole slaw, noodles/lemon no drink

Dinner: ate out hamburger lettuce tomato cheese, onion rings, 21 ounces soda

Treatment Day filling tired going in after coming home very tired and had headache

79.4KG going in after 76.7

17th

Breakfast: 3 eggs 1 cup of oak brand hot cereal, 21 ounces coffee

Lunch: turkey sandwich, lettuce tomato cheese, 16 ounces soda

Dinner: burrito, 16 ounces soda

No Treatment little tired some energy

18th

Breakfast: 1 bowl cold cereal, 21 ounces coffee

Lunch: renal meal: glazed chicken bites, Mexican zucchini/corn white rice no drink

Dinner: renal meal: fish/lemon/tarragon sauce, lemon rice green beans 16 ounces soda

Treatment day I have some energy be for going in/coming filling great have lot of energy

Be for 79.6 KG after 76.5 KG

19th

Breakfast: skipped

Lunch: salad, turkey sandwich, 16 ounces soda

Dinner: rice, chicken salad, 16 ounces soda

20th

Breakfast: 3 eggs 1 cup of oak brand hot cereal, 21 ounces coffee

Lunch: renal meal: Chicken Fajitas, Tortilla Corn Niblets/Se, no drink

Dinner: renal meal: bow pie pasta/turkey/vegg, green bean, crisp,

Treatment day felt great be for and after

Be for 79.6 KG after 76.5 KG

21st

Breakfast: skipped

Lunch blueberry muffin, 21 ounces soda , ate out

Dinner: Hotdog, chips, salad

No Treatment had a sleepless night very tired

22nd

Breakfast: 3 eggs 1 cup of oak brand hot cereal, 3 sausage, 21 ounces coffee

Lunch: skipped

Dinner: ate out hamburger lettuce tomato cheese, onion rings, 21 ounces soda

No Treatment some energy not tired

23rd

Breakfast: 3 eggs 1 cup of oak brand hot cereal, 3 sausage, 21 ounces coffee

Lunch: renal meal: pasta primavera/turkey, asparagus, green peas

Dinner: BBQ chicken, rice, veg, 21 ounces water

Treatment day filling ok be for going in after coming home im a little tired

78.3 KG be for going in, coming home 76.5 KG

24th

Breakfast: 2 eggs, 3 sausage, 2 toast, 3 cups of 21 ounces coffee ate out

Lunch: ate out hamburger lettuce tomato cheese, fries, 2, 21 ounces soda

Dinner: renal meal Italian pasta/vegetables, summer squash medley, green beans, 21 ounces soda

No Treatment felted good in tell the afternoon then very tired after that

25th

Breakfast: 3 eggs 1 cup of oak brand hot cereal, 3 sausage, 21 ounces coffee

Lunch: renal meal: meatball stroganoff/white g, noodles/lemon, peas/carrots, no drink

Dinner: Renal meal: Cajun hamburger, green peas 2, 21 ounces soda

Treatment day felt good going in and coming home some energy

77.9KG going in 76.5 KG after Treatment

26th

Breakfast: 3 eggs 1 cup of oak brand hot cereal, 3 sausage, 21 ounces coffee

Lunch: pizza, 21 ounces soda

Dinner: hotdog, chips, and 21 ounces soda

No Treatment a little tried, some energy

27th

Breakfast: 3 eggs 1 cup of oak brand hot cereal, 3 sausage, 21 ounces coffee

Lunch: Renal Meal: sausage spaghetti, parmesan zucchini green peas, no drink

Dinner: Renal Meal: meatloaf/BBQ glaze, noodles, peas/carrots 21 ounces water

Treatment day felt tiered all day

78.7KG going in 76.5KG after Treatment

28th

Breakfast: 3 eggs 1 cup of oak brand hot cereal, 3 sausage, 21 ounces coffee

Lunch: ate out 2 hamburger lettuce tomato cheese, 21 ounces water

Dinner: BBQ chicken, steak, pasta/vegetables salad, 2 beers 21 ounces

No Treatment felted well had some energy the whole day

29th

Breakfast: 1 cup of oak brand hot cereal, 21 ounces coffee

Lunch: turkey sandwich lettuce tomato cheese, 21 ounces water

Dinner: spaghetti, Turkey, chicken 21 ounces water

No Treatment felted well had some energy the whole day

30th

Breakfast: skipped

Lunch: renal meal: chicken fajitas, tortilla, corn niblets/se no drink

Dinner: oven fried chicken, carrots/dill, corn 21 ounces water

 Treatment day some energy be for going in 78.0 KG

A little tired coming home 76.5KG

31st

Breakfast: 1 cup of oak brand hot cereal, 21 ounces coffee

Lunch: spaghetti, Turkey, chicken, 21 ounces water, soda ounces soda

Dinner: ate out hamburger, onion rings, 21 ounces soda

No Treatment felted well had lots of energy the whole day

Web sites

Fundraising

HelpHopeLive.org

They're a nonprofit organization that helps people with major medical needs help fundraise (and it's tax-deductible

Nft.org

will help you with fund raising ideas and gives you a tax free place to save for transplant related expenses.

Education

Kidneyschool.org

http://www.kidney-cares.org

http://www.nephinc.com

www.kidney.org   The National Kidney Foundation

http://www.davita.com they have Class and Videos

I typed in the Search for this Understanding Your Lab Work

http://www.davita.com/kidney-disease/overview/symptoms-and-diagnosis/understanding-your-lab-work/e/4724

http://kidney.niddk.nih.gov

What is dialysis? What is kidney dialysis?

http://cancerfactscentral.org/what-is-dialysis-what-is-kidney-dialysis/

This Talk about both Hemodialysis and Peritoneal

http://viralfactsfactory.com/how-haemodialysis-and-peritoneal-dialysis-are-performed/

Support group

http://www.igan.ca

All so check out Facebook, yahoo & google groups

https://sites.google.com/site/kidneycrowd

Food

http://www.wrha.mb.ca/prog/nutrition/files/dialysis_cookbook.pdf

http://ww38.nstyleid.com/

Renal meals

http://www.councilonaging.com/therapeutic-renal-meals-save-lives-of-all-ages/

Other

UCF Medical Center for Transplantation Evaluation

http://www.ucsfhealth.org/conditions/kidney_transplant/diagnosis.html

http://www.kidneybuzz.com/fistula1/

This site is for incompatible donor, to help them find a match

http://www.kidneymatch.org/

http://www.ssa.gov/work/

Necklaces or bracelets

https://www.hopepaige.com/

Watchtower bible and track society of Pennsylvania

For more information other subject of interest please go to JW.org

http://preventionandwellness.net/top-10-symptoms-of-kidney-disease-that-you-need-to-know-2/

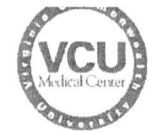

The Renal Diet

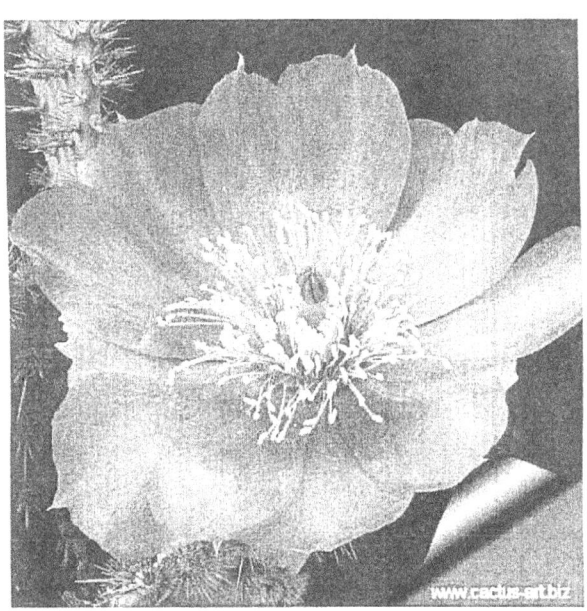

www.cactus-art.biz

A Guide to Eating Healthier
for Hemodialysis Patients

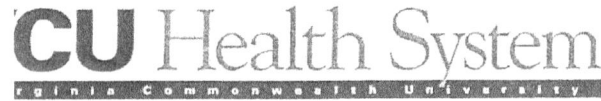

CU Health System
Virginia Commonwealth University

MCV Hospitals and Physicians

Controlling Your Phosphorus

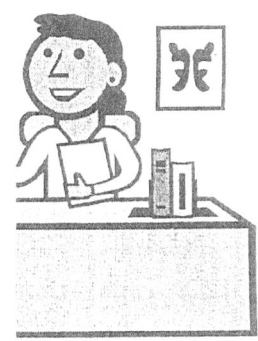 Phosphorus is a mineral that healthy kidneys get rid of in the urine. In kidneys that are failing, phosphorus builds up in the blood and may cause many problems including muscle aches and pains, brittle, easily broken bones, calcification of the heart, skin, joints, and blood vessels. To keep your phosphorus levels in check, consider the following tips:

. Limit high phosphorus foods such as:
- Meats, poultry, dairy and fish (you should have 1 serving of 7-8 ounces)
- Milk and other dairy products like cheese (you should have one 4 oz. serving)

2. Avoid high phosphorus foods such as:
- Lima Beans, Black Beans, Red Beans, Black-eyed Peas, White Beans, and Garbanzo Beans
- Dark, whole or unrefined grains
- Refrigerator doughs like Pillsbury
- Dried vegetables and fruits
- Chocolate
- Dark colored sodas

3. Don't forget to take your phosphate binders with meals and snacks.
- Your doctor will prescribe a medication called a phosphate binder which will be some type of polymer gel or calcium medication. You need to take your phosphate binder as prescribed by your doctor. Often you will take a phosphate binder with every meal and snack.

4. Usually your diet is limited to 1000 mg of phosphorus per day.

Controlling Your Potassium

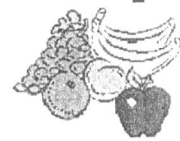 Potassium is an element that is necessary for the body to keep a normal water balance between the cells and body fluids. All foods contain some potassium, but some contain larger amounts.

Normal kidney function will remove potassium through urination. Kidneys that are not functioning properly cannot remove the potassium in the urine, so it builds up in the blood. This can be *very* dangerous to your heart. High potassium can cause irregular heart beats and can even cause the heart to stop if the potassium levels get to high.

Typically, there are no symptoms for someone with a high potassium level. If you are concerned about your potassium level, check with your doctor, and follow the tips below.

- Usually a renal patient's diet should be limited to 2000 mg of potassium each day.

- The following foods are high in potassium:

Bananas	Avocado	Oranges
Orange Juice	Prunes	Prune Juice
Tomatoes	Tomato Juice	Tomato Sauce
Cantaloupe	Tomato Puree	Honeydew Melon
Nuts	Papaya	Chocolate
Red Beans	Milk	White Beans
Lima Beans	Garbanzo Beans	Black Beans
Lentils	Split peas	Baked Beans

Specially Prepared Potatoes:
1. Peel and slice into 1/8 inch pieces.
2. Soak 1 cup potatoes in 5 cups of water for 2 hours.
3. Drain and rinse and drain.
4. Cook in a large amount of water.
5. Drain and mash, fry or serve plain.

Controlling Your Sodium

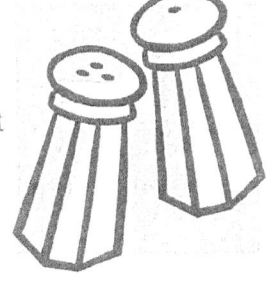

Sodium, or sodium chloride is an element that is used by all living creatures to regulate the water content in the body. Usually a sodium restriction comes in the form of "No Added Salt." This is necessary because a greater intake of sodium will result in poorly controlled blood pressure and excessive thirst which can lead to difficulty adhering to the fluid restrictions in your diet.

To limit your sodium, you should:

- Avoid table salt and any seasonings that end with the word "salt"

- Avoid salt substitutes (they contain potassium)

- Avoid salty meats such as bacon, ham, sausage, hot dogs, lunch meats, canned meats, or bologna

- Avoid salty snacks such as cheese curls, salted crackers, nuts, and chips

- Avoid canned soups, frozen dinners, and instant noodles

- Avoid bottled sauces, pickles, olives, and MSG

Controlling Your Protein

Protein is important to aid in growth and maintenance of body tissue. Protein also plays a role in fighting infection, healing of wounds, and provides a source of energy to the body.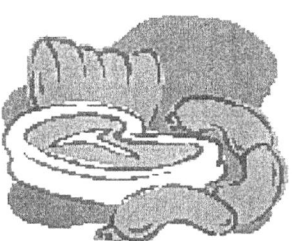

- You should make sure to eat 7-8 ounces of protein every day. Foods that are high in protein include beef, pork, veal, chicken, turkey, fish, seafood, and eggs.

- 1 egg is equal to 1 ounce of protein, and three ounces of protein is comparable to the size of a deck of cards.

Controlling Your Fluid Intake

People on dialysis often have decreased urine output, so increased fluid in the body can put unnecessary pressure on the person's heart and lungs.

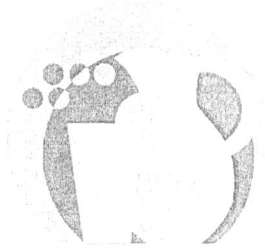

- A fluid allowance for individual patients is calculated on the basis of 'urine plus 500ml.' The 500 ml covers the loss of fluids through the skin and lungs.

- Most patients will not urinate as much once they begin Hemodialysis. Those who produce a lot of urine may be able to drink more than those who do not produce urine.

- Between each dialysis treatment, patients are expected to gain a little weight due to the water content in foods (fruits and vegetables).

- The amount of fluid in a typical day's meal (excluding fluids such as water, tea, etc.) is at least 500 ml and therefore expected daily weight gain is between 0.4 – 0.5kg.

- To control fluid intake, patients should:

  ❑ Not drink more than what your doctor orders (usually 4 cups of fluid each day)

  ❑ Count all foods that will melt at room temperature as fluids (Jell-O® , popsicles, and fruit ices).

Grocery List Suggestions

Meat/Protein Foods
- Beef
- Chicken
- Egg Substitute (Egg Beaters®, Scramblers®)
- Eggs
- Fish
- Lamb
- Pork (fresh) (pork chops, roast)
- Shellfish
- Tofu (soft)
- Tuna (canned in water)
- Turkey
- Veal
- Wild Game

Fruits
(Serving size = 1 medium-size fruit or 1/2 cup canned, no added sugar)
- Apple Juice
- Apples
- Applesauce
- Apricot Nectar
- Apricots (canned)
- Blackberries
- Cherries
- Cranberries
- Cranberry Juice
- Cranberry Sauce
- Figs (fresh)
- Fruit Cocktail
- Grapefruit
- Grape Juice
- Grapes
- Lemon
- Lemon Juice
- Lime
- Lime Juice
- Loganberries
- Lychees
- Peach (canned)
- Peach nectar
- Pear nectar
- Pears (canned)
- Pineapple
- Plums
- Raspberries
- Strawberries
- Tangerines

Vegetables
(Serving size = 1/2 cup, no added salt)
- Alfalfa Sprouts
- Arugula
- Asparagus
- Bean sprouts
- Beets (canned)
- Cabbage (green, red)
- Carrots
- Cauliflower
- Celery
- Chayote
- Chili peppers
- Chives
- Coleslaw
- Corn
- Cucumber
- Eggplant
- Endive
- Garlic
- Gingerroot
- Green beans
- Hominy
- Jalapeños (fresh)
- Kale
- Leeks
- Lettuce
- Mixed Vegetables
- Mushrooms
- Onions
- Parsley
- Peas (English)
- Pimentos
- Radicchio
- Radishes
- Seaweed kelp
- Spaghetti Squash
- Summer squash (scallop, crookneck, straightneck, zucchini)
- Sweet Peppers (green, red, yellow)
- Tomatillos
- Turnips
- Turnip Greens
- Water Chestnuts
- Watercress
- Yambean (jicama), cooked

Breads/Cereals/Grains
- Bagels (plain, blueberry, egg, raisin)
- Bread (white, French, Italian, rye, soft wheat)
- Bread sticks (plain)
- Cereals, dry, low salt (Corn Pops®, Cocoa Puffs®, Sugar Smacks®, Fruity Pebbles®, Puffed Wheat®, Puffed Rice®)
- Cereals cooked (Cream of Rice®, or Wheat, Farina®, Malt-o-meal®)
- Couscous
- Crackers (unsalted)
- Dinner rolls or hard rolls
- English muffins
- Grits
- Hamburger/hot dog buns
- Macaroni
- Melba toast
- Noodles
- Oyster crackers
- Pita bread
- Popcorn (unsalted)
- Pretzels (unsalted)
- Rice (brown, white)
- Rice cakes (apple-cinnamon, etc)
- Spaghetti
- Tortillas (flour)

Dairy/Dairy Substitutes
- Nondairy creamers
- Nondairy frozen dessert topping (Cool Whip®)
- Nondairy frozen desserts (Mocha Mix®)
- Rice milk, unfortified

Beverages
(Keep in mind your fluid restriction) (Diabetics – use caution for sugar intake) (Regular or diet)
- 7-Up
- Cherry 7-Up®
- Cream Soda
- Ginger ale
- Grape soda
- Lemon-lime soda
- Mellow Yellow®
- Mountain Dew®
- Orange soda
- Root Beer
- Slice®
- Sprite®
- Coffee
- Fruit Punch
- Hi-C® (Cherry, grape)
- Horchata®
- Juices (apple, cranberry, grape)
- Kool-Aid®
- Lemonade or Limeade
- Mineral Water
- Nectars (apricot, peach, pear, 1/2 cup serving)
- Nondairy creamers (Coffee Rich®, Mocha Mix®, etc.)
- Sunny Delight® (citrus flavor)
- Tea

Fats
- Butter
- Cream Cheese
- Margarine
- Mayonnaise
- Miracle Whip®
- Nondairy creamers
- Salad Dressings
- Sour Cream
- Vegetable oils (preferably canola or olive oil)

Grocery List Suggestions

Seasonings and Spices

- ❑ Allspice
- ❑ Basil
- ❑ Bay leaf
- ❑ Caraway seed
- ❑ Chives
- ❑ Cilantro
- ❑ Cinnamon
- ❑ Cloves
- ❑ Cumin
- ❑ Curry
- ❑ Dill
- ❑ Extracts (almond, lemon, lime, maple, orange, peppermint, vanilla, walnut)
- ❑ Fennel
- ❑ Garlic powder
- ❑ Ginger
- ❑ Horseradish (root)
- ❑ Lemon Juice
- ❑ Mrs. Dash®
- ❑ Nutmeg
- ❑ Onion powder or flakes
- ❑ Oregano
- ❑ Paprika
- ❑ Parsley or parsley flakes
- ❑ Pepper (ground)
- ❑ Pimentos
- ❑ Poppy seed
- ❑ Rosemary
- ❑ Saccharin
- ❑ Saffron
- ❑ Sage
- ❑ Savory
- ❑ Sesame seeds
- ❑ Tarragon
- ❑ Thyme
- ❑ Turmeric
- ❑ Vinegar

Desserts/Snacks/Sweets
(Diabetics – use caution)

- ❑ Animal Crackers
- ❑ Cake (angel food, butter, lemon, pound, spice, strawberry, white, yellow)
- ❑ Candy corn
- ❑ Chewing gum
- ❑ Cinnamon drops
- ❑ Cookies (ginger snaps, shortbread, sugar, vanilla wafers)
- ❑ Corn cakes
- ❑ Cotton Candy
- ❑ Doughnuts
- ❑ Fruit ice
- ❑ Graham crackers
- ❑ Gumdrops
- ❑ Gummy Bears ®
- ❑ Hard candy
- ❑ Hot Tamale® candy
- ❑ Jell-O®
- ❑ Jelly beans
- ❑ Jolly Ranchers®
- ❑ LifeSavers®
- ❑ Lollipops
- ❑ Marshmallows
- ❑ Newtons® (fig. strawberry, apple, blueberry)
- ❑ Pie (apple, berry, cherry, lemon, peach)

Other
(Diabetics– use with caution)

- ❑ Apple Butter
- ❑ Corn syrup
- ❑ Honey
- ❑ Jam
- ❑ Jelly
- ❑ Maple Syrup
- ❑ Marmalade
- ❑ Powdered sugar
- ❑ Sugar, brown or white

Notes

_____
_____
_____
_____
_____
_____
_____
_____
_____
_____
_____
_____
_____
_____
_____
_____
_____
_____
_____
_____
_____
_____
_____
_____
_____
_____
_____
_____
_____
_____
_____
_____
_____
_____
_____
_____

Fast Food Facts for the Renal Patient

By Maria Karalis, MBA, RD, LD

Quick-service restaurants provide us with a quick, easy, inexpensive bite when we're pressed for time. Americans love fast food and there are so many items to choose from! A lot of chains are now offering lower-fat options and if chosen wisely, fast foods can be healthy AND fit into your renal diet.

If you are a regular through the drive-up window or frequently dine in at fast food restaurants, keep these tips in mind.

Some Ordering Tips:

- Burgers and sandwiches are high in sodium because they are pre-salted. This may be difficult for the quick-service restaurant to omit the salt. Be sure to ask before you order.

- Remember that fries and baked potatoes are rich in potassium. But if you can't imagine a burger without the fries, order a small serving and ask for unsalted, if possible.

- Keep in mind that catsup, mustard, and pickles are all high in sodium. Keep condiments, special sauces and dressings to a minimum. Request that these toppings be served "on the side" so you can control the amount.

- Beverage sizes typically are large or "super-size" and can contribute to fluid overload if the entire beverage is consumed. Order a small beverage and be sure to count it as part of your fluid allowance.

- Balance fast food items with other food choices. As you order, consider the other foods you have eaten or will eat during the day.

- Choose broiled, steamed or grilled items over deep fat fried foods. To trim the fat from fried items, order the regular variety instead of the extra crispy and remove the skin before eating. Removing the skin also lowers the sodium content since most batters and coatings usually include seasonings rich in sodium.

The huge variety of vegetables and fruits can provide you with vitamins A and C, folic acid and fiber. Be careful though, a trip to the salad bar can provide you with more fat and calories than a burger and fries! There are many salad bar items that can easily fit into your renal diet. Below is a list of items to assist you in choosing sensibly from any salad bar.

Fast Food Facts continued...

Include these items in your salad bar choices:

Alfalfa Sprouts	Gelatin salads	Oil and vinegar dressing
Beets	Green beans	Okra
Cauliflower	Green peas	Onions
Celery sticks	Green peppers	Parmesan cheese
Chinese Noodles	Italian, low calorie dressing	Radishes
Cole Slaw	Lettuce, escarole, endive	Tuna in spring water
Cucumbers	Macaroni salad	Vinaigrette or low fat
Eggs, chopped	Mushrooms	Zucchini

Limit these items in your salad bar choices:

Avocado	Nuts	Sunflower seeds
Bacon Bits	Olives	Shredded cheddar cheese
Chickpeas	Pickles	Thick salad dressings
Chow mein noodles	Potato Salad	Three-bean salads
Fried bread croutons	Raisins	Tomatoes
Kidney Beans	Relishes	

Do you know what you are eating?

Get a breakdown of fat, calories and other nutrition information (potassium, phosphorus or sodium) from the store manager. You can also check out the restaurant's website for a complete nutritional analysis of all their menu items. Please note that obtaining information on potassium and phosphorus can be difficult, since these values are not required by the US Department of Agriculture on food labels. The following table provides you with the nutritional analysis of some fast food menu items to help you make educated choices.

Note the serving size and work with your renal dietitian to safely add these menu items into your eating plan.

Many Items are loaded with sodium so limit your sodium intake for the rest of the day. Watch your fluid intake because these foods will make you more thirsty than usual. Some items may require that you increase your dose of phosphate binders.

My Recommendations:
- McDonalds®: plain hamburger on a bun
- Burger King®: plain hamburger on a bun or BK Broiler, plain
- Taco Bell®: taco, limit the tomatoes
- Wendy's®: single hamburger or grilled chicken sandwich, plain

www.ingramcontent.com/pod-product-compliance
Lightning Source LLC
Chambersburg PA
CBHW082305200526
45168CB00018B/3416